CW00572212

Mediterranean Diet Snack Recipes

50 Simple and Tasty *Recipes to* Eat *Fresh, Cook Simple, and Live Clean*

Maria Greenwood

Table of Contents

Introduction

The Basics of the Mediterranean Diet

The foods that we eat have been known to contribute greatly to how our health turns out. Feeding on unhealthy foods is known to cause a myriad of health issues, including chronic diseases; therefore, the diet that one adopts should be given a lot of emphasis. The Mediterranean diet is considered as one of the world's healthiest diet. It's an eating approach that puts emphasis on eating whole foods that are full of flavor. It's a diet that is abundant in fruits, whole grains, vegetables, legumes and olive oil. The diet also features lean sources of protein, and the red wine is consumed in moderate amounts.

The Mediterranean diet is also one of the top most popular diets, and it's not the type of diet where the end goal is only to lose weight; it's considered more of a lifestyle. It should be adopted as a daily practice and a way of living that's sustainable. The Mediterranean diet incorporates traditional and healthy living habits of people from the countries that border the Mediterranean Sea, such as Greece, Italy, France, Spain, Morocco and the like.

The diet varies by country and the region it is adopted, so it may have a range of definitions. However, it is a diet with high intake of vegetables, legumes, fruits, nuts, beans, grains, unsaturated fats like olive oil and fish among others. It, however, includes lower intake of dairy foods and meat. There are several benefits that have been associated with the Mediterranean diet, such as good health and a healthier heart.

Various research studies have proven that those who put a lot of emphasis on healthy fats, whole grains and fish not only weigh less but also experience decreased risks of heart-related diseases, dementia and depression.

Eating in this way means that one gets little room for consuming the unhealthy junk and processed foods, which normally lead to being overweight and obese

Benefits of the Mediterranean Diet

1. Boosts Your Brain Health. Preserve memory and prevent cognitive decline by following a Mediterranean diet that will limit processed foods, refined bread, and red meats. Have a glassof wine versus hard liquor.

2. Decreases Risks for Type 2 Diabetes. It can help stabilize blood sugar while protecting against type 2 diabetes with its low-carb elements. The Med diet maintains a richness in fiber, which will digest slowly while preventing variances in your blood sugar. It also can help you maintain a healthier weight, which is another trigger for diabetes.

3. Suggests Improvement for Those with Parkinson's Disease. By consuming foods on the Mediterranean diet, you add high levels of antioxidants that can prevent your body from undergoing oxidative stress, which is a damaging process that will attack your cells. The menu plan can reduce your risk factors in half.

4. Improves Poor Eyesight. Older individuals suffer from poor eyesight, but in many cases, the Mediterranean diet has provided notable improvement. An Australian Center for EyeResearch discovered that the individuals who consumed a minimum of 100 ml (0.42 cup) of olive oil weekly were almost 50% less likely to develop macular degeneration versus those who ate less than one ml each week.

5. Helps to Reduce the Risk of Heart Disease. The New England Journal of Medicine provided evidence in 2013 from a randomized clinical trial. The trial was implemented in Spain, whereas individuals did not have cardiovascular disease at enrollment but were in the 'high risk' category. The incidence of major cardiovascular events was reduced by the Mediterranean diet that was supplemented with extra-virgin olive oil or nuts. In one study, men who consumed fish in this manner reduced the risk by 23% of death from heart disease.

6. The Risk of Alzheimer's Disease Is Reduced. In 2018, the journal Neurology studied 70 brain scans of individuals who had no signs of dementia at the onset. They followed the eating patterns in a two-year study resulting in individuals who were on the Med diet had a lesser increase of the depots and reduced energy use — potentially signaling risk for Alzheimer's.

7. Helps Lessen the Risk of Some Types of Cancer. According to the results of a group study, the diet is associated with a lessened risk of stomach cancer (gastric adenocarcinoma).

1. Cucumber Sandwich Bites

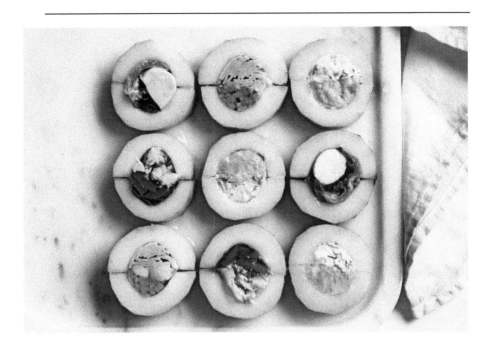

Preparation Time: 5 minutes

Cooking Time: 0 minutes

Servings: 12

Ingredients:

- One cucumber, sliced
- Eight slices of whole wheat bread
- Two tablespoons cream cheese, soft
- One tablespoon chive, chopped
- ¼ cup avocado, peeled, pitted, and mashed
- One teaspoon mustard

- Salt and black pepper to the taste

Directions:

1. Spread the mashed avocado on each bread slice.

2. Also, spread the rest of the ingredients except the cucumber slices.

3. Divide the cucumber slices into the bread slices.

4. Cut each slice in thirds, arrange on a platter and serve.

Nutrition:

Calories: 187 Fat: 12.4g Fiber: 2.1g Carbohydrates: 4.5g Protein: 8.2g

2. Summer Squash Ribbons with Lemon and Ricotta

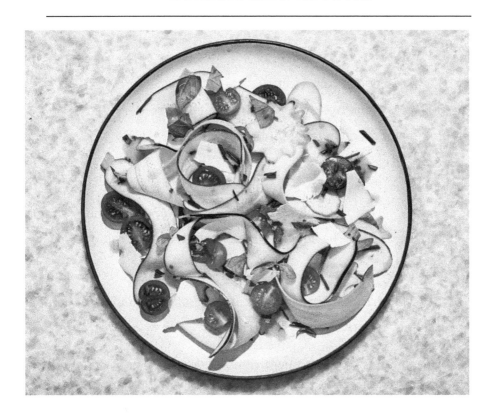

Preparation Time: 20 minutes

Cooking Time: 0 minutes

Servings: 4

Ingredients:

- Two medium zucchini or yellow squash
- ½ cup ricotta cheese

- Two tablespoons fresh mint, chopped, plus additional mint
- leaves for garnish
- Two tablespoons fresh parsley, chopped
- Zest of ½ lemon
- Two teaspoons lemon juice
- ½ teaspoon kosher salt
- ¼ teaspoon freshly ground black pepper
- One tablespoon extra-virgin olive oil

Directions:

1. Using a vegetable peeler, make ribbons by peeling the summer squash lengthwise. The squash ribbons will resemble the wide pasta, pappardelle.

2. In a bowl, mix the ricotta cheese, mint, parsley, lemon zest, lemon juice, salt, and black pepper.

3. Place mounds of the squash ribbons evenly on four plates, then dollop the ricotta mixture on top. Sprinkle with the olive oil, then garnish with the mint leaves.

Nutrition:

Calories: 90 Total Fat: 6g Cholesterol: 10mg Total Carbohydrates: 5g

Fiber: 1g

3. Green Beans with Pine Nuts and Garlic

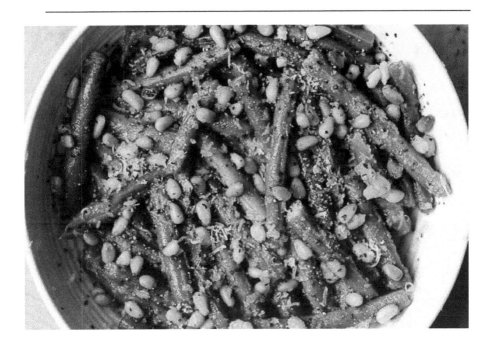

Preparation Time: 10 minutes

Cooking Time: 20 minutes

Servings: 4 to 6

Ingredients:

- 1-pound green beans, trimmed
- One head garlic (10 to 12 cloves), smashed
- Two tablespoons extra-virgin olive oil
- ½ teaspoon kosher salt
- ¼ teaspoon red pepper flakes

13

- One tablespoon white wine vinegar
- ¼ cup pine nuts, toasted

Directions:

1. Preheat the oven to 425°F.

2. In a large bowl, blend the green beans, garlic, olive oil, salt, and red pepper flakes and mix—put it in a single layer on the baking sheet. Roast for 10 minutes, stir, and roast for another 10 minutes, or until golden brown.

3. Mix the cooked green beans with the vinegar and top with the pine nuts.

Nutrition:

Calories: 165 Total Fat: 13g Total Carbohydrates: 12g Fiber: 4g

Sugars: 4g Protein: 4g

4. Cucumbers with Feta, Mint, and Sumac

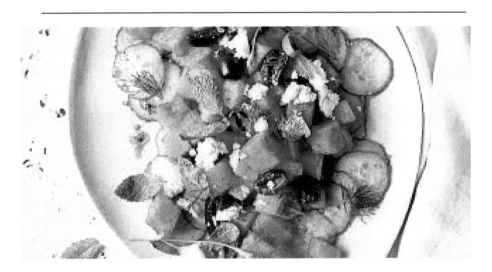

Preparation Time: 15 minutes

Cooking Time: 0 minutes

Servings: 4

Ingredients:

- One tablespoon extra-virgin olive oil
- One tablespoon lemon juice
- Two teaspoons ground sumac
- ½ teaspoon kosher salt
- Two hothouse or English cucumbers, diced
- ¼ cup crumbled feta cheese
- One tablespoon fresh mint, chopped

- One tablespoon fresh parsley, chopped
- 1/8 teaspoon red pepper flakes

Directions:

1. In a bowl, whisk together the lemon juice, olive oil, sumac, and salt. Add the cucumber and feta cheese and toss well.

2. Transfer to a serving dish and sprinkle with mint, parsley, and red pepper flakes.

Nutrition:

Calories: 85 Total Fat: 6g Cholesterol: 8mg Total Carbohydrates: 8g

Fiber: 1g Protein: 4g

5. Cherry Tomato Bruschetta

Preparation Time: 15 minutes

Servings: 4

- Ingredients:
- 8 ounces assorted cherry tomatoes, halved
- 1/3 cup fresh herbs, chopped (such as basil, parsley, tarragon,
- dill)
- One tablespoon extra-virgin olive oil
- ¼ teaspoon kosher salt
- 1/8 teaspoon freshly ground black pepper
- ¼ cup ricotta cheese
- Four slices whole-wheat bread, toasted

Directions:

1. Combine the tomatoes, herbs, olive oil, salt, and black pepper in a medium bowl and mix gently.

2. Spread one tablespoon of ricotta cheese onto each slice of toast—spoon one-quarter of the tomato mixture onto each bruschetta. If desired, garnish with more herbs.

Nutrition:

Calories: 100 Total Fat: 6g Cholesterol: 5mg Total Carbohydrates: 10g

Fiber: 2g Protein: 4g

6. Roasted Rosemary Olives

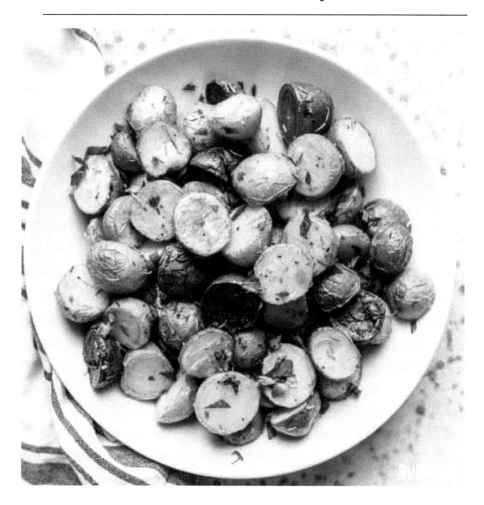

Preparation Time: 5 minutes

Cooking Time: 25 minutes

Servings: 4

Ingredients:

- 1 cup mixed variety olives, pitted and rinsed
- Two tablespoons lemon juice
- One tablespoon extra-virgin olive oil
- Six garlic cloves, peeled
- Four rosemary sprigs

Directions:

1. Preheat the oven to 400°F.

2. Combine the olive oil, olives, lemon juice, and garlic in a medium bowl and mix.

3. Spread in a single layer on the prepared baking sheet. Sprinkle on the rosemary—roast for 25 minutes, tossing halfway through.

4. Take away the rosemary leaves from the stem and place them in a serving bowl. Add the olives and mix before serving.

Nutrition:

Calories: 100 Total Fat: 9g Cholesterol: 0mg Total Carbohydrates: 4g

Protein: 0g

7. Spiced Maple Nuts

Preparation Time: 5 minutes Cooking Time: 10 minutes Servings: 2

Ingredients:

- 2 cups raw walnuts or pecans
- One teaspoon extra-virgin olive oil
- One teaspoon ground sumac
- ½ teaspoon pure maple syrup
- ¼ teaspoon kosher salt
- ¼ teaspoon ground ginger
- 2 to 4 rosemary sprigs

Directions:

1. Preheat the oven to 350°F.

2. In a bowl, combine the nuts, olive oil, sumac, maple syrup, salt, ginger, mix. Spread in a sole layer on the prepared baking sheet. Add the rosemary. Roast for 8 to 10 minutes, or wait until golden and fragrant.

3. Remove the rosemary leaves from the stems and place them in a serving bowl. Add the nuts and toss to combine before serving.

Nutrition:

Calories: 175

Total Fat: 18g Cholesterol: 0mg Total Carbohydrates: 4g Protein: 3g

8. Figs with Mascarpone and Honey

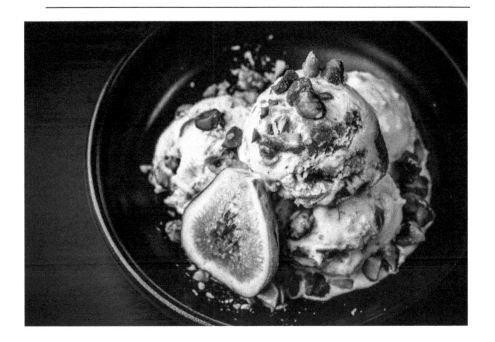

Preparation Time: 5 minutes

Cooking Time: 5 minutes

Servings: 4

Ingredients:

- 1/3 cup walnuts, chopped
- Eight fresh figs halved
- ¼ cup mascarpone cheese
- One tablespoon honey
- ¼ teaspoon flaked sea salt

Directions:

1. In a frypan with medium heat, toast the walnuts, often stirring, for 3 to 5 minutes.

2. Arrange the figs cut-side up on a plate or platter. Using your finger, create a small depression in each fig's cut side and fill with mascarpone cheese. Sprinkle with a bit of the walnut, drizzle with the honey, and add a tiny pinch of sea salt.

Nutrition:

Calories: 200 Total Fat: 13g Cholesterol: 18mg Total Carbohydrates: 24g Protein: 3g

9. Pistachio-Stuffed Dates

Preparation Time: 10 minutes

Cooking Time: 0 minutes

Servings: 4

Ingredients:

- ½ cup unsalted pistachios shelled
- ¼ teaspoon kosher salt
- 8 Medjool dates, pitted

Directions:

1. In a food processor, add the salt and pistachios. Process until combined to chunky nut butter, 3 to 5 minutes.

2. Split open the dates and spoon the pistachio nut butter into each half.

Nutrition:

Calories: 220 Total Fat: 7g Cholesterol: 0mg Total Carbohydrates: 41g

Protein: 4g

10.   Portable Packed Picnic Pieces

Preparation Time: 10 minutes

Cooking Time: 0 minutes

Servings: 1

Ingredients:

- 1-slice of whole-wheat bread, cut into bite-size pieces
- 10-pcs cherry tomatoes
- ¼-oz. aged cheese, sliced
- 6-pcs oil-cured olives

Directions:

1. Pack each of the ingredients in a portable container to serve

you while snacking on the go.

Nutrition:

Calories: 197 Total Fats: 9g Fiber: 4g Carbohydrates: 22g Protein: 7g

11.   Mediterranean Picnic Snack

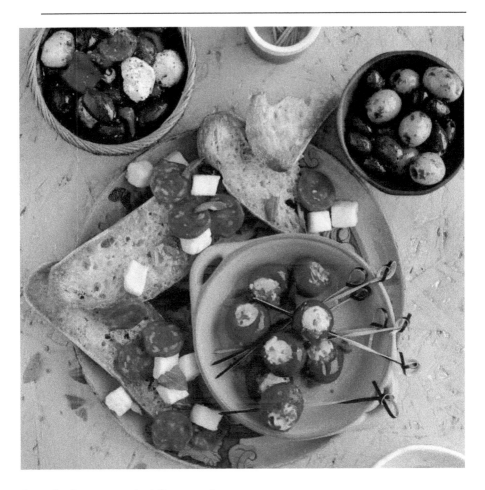

(Total Time: 10 min | Serves 2)

Ingredients

- Crusty whole-wheat bread – 1 slice
- Cherry tomatoes – 10
- Oil-cured olives – 6
- Sliced aged cheese – ¼ ounce

Instructions

Combine the bread pieces, cheese, tomatoes and olives into a portable container.

Serve and enjoy.

Nutrition Information:

Calories per serving: 197; Carbohydrates: 22g; Protein: 7g; Fat: 9g; Sugar: 0g; Sodium: 454mg; Fiber: 1g

12. Tomato and Basil Finger Sandwiches

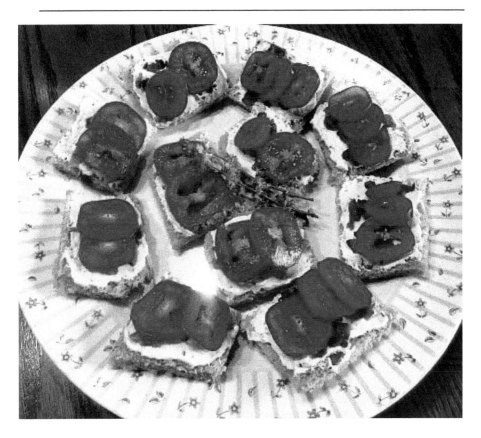

(Total Time: 15 min | Serves 4)

Ingredients

- Whole-wheat bread – 4 slices
- Mayonnaise – 8 teaspoons
- Tomato thick slices – 4
- Freshly ground pepper – 1/8 teaspoon

- Salt – 1/8 teaspoon
- Sliced fresh basil – 4 teaspoons

Instructions

1. Cut bread into rounds that are larger than tomato and then spread each with mayonnaise.
2. Top it with tomatoes, basil, salt and pepper.

Nutrition Information:

Calories per serving: 85; Carbohydrates: 13g; Protein: 3g; Fat: 3g; Sugar: 2g; Sodium:324mg; Fiber: 1g

13. Greek Yoghurt with Strawberries

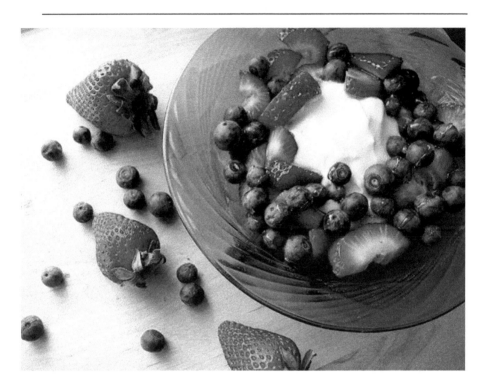

(Total Time: 10 min | Serves 2)

Ingredients

- Nonfat plain Greek yoghurt – ½ cup
- Sliced fresh strawberries – ½ cup

Instructions

1. Place yoghurt in a bowl and then top with the strawberries.

Nutrition Information:

Calories per serving: 80; Carbohydrates: 7g; Protein: 12g; Fat: 1g;
Sugar: 4g; Sodium:130mg; Fiber: 2g

14.   Herbed Olives

(Total Time: 20 min | Serves 4)

Ingredients

- Favorite olives – 3 cups
- Olive oils – 2 teaspoons
- Dried oregano – 1/8 teaspoon
- Dried basil – 1/8 teaspoon
- Crushed clove garlic – 1
- Freshly ground pepper to taste

Instructions

Toss the olives, basil, garlic, oregano and pepper into a medium bowl.

Nutrition Information:

Calories per serving: 47; Carbohydrates: 1g; Protein: 0g; Fat: 5g; Sugar: 0g; Sodium:224mg; Fiber: 1g

15.   Bacon-Wrapped Chicken Tenders

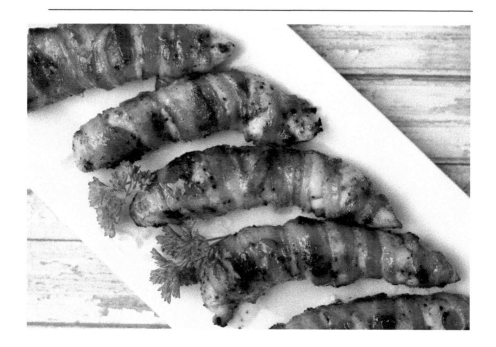

(Total Time: 25 min| Serves 4)

Ingredients

- Chicken breast tenderloins – 1 lb
- Bacon slices – 8
- Cheddar cheese – 4 slices

Instructions

1. Fill a bowl with water and then add salt. Add the chicken breasts and then allow to stay in the water for 10 minutes.

2. Get the oven preheated to 4500F and then line baking sheet with parchment paper.

3. Remove chicken from the water and then pat to dry. Place a piece of cheese over each chicken piece and wrap together in bacon slice.

4. Place the wrapped chicken on a baking sheet with the cheese side up.

5. Repeat with the remaining cheese, chicken and bacon. Bake for 16 minutes or until the chicken is well cooked.

6. Place it under a broiler for a few minutes until bacon is crisp.

7. Serve and enjoy.

Nutrition Information:

Calories per serving: 301; Carbohydrates: 1g; Protein: 25g; Fat: 17g; Sugar: 0g; Sodium:210mg; Fiber: 0g

16.   Sweet and Spicy Meat Balls

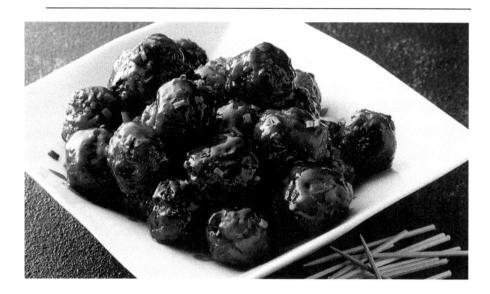

(Total Time: 30 min| Serves 6)

Ingredients

- Cooked meatballs – 16 oz
- Crushed red pepper – ½ tablespoon
- Cayenne pepper – ½ teaspoon
- Grape jelly – 12 ounce
- Water – 1 cup
- Chopped green onions for garnish

Instructions

1. Add the cooked meatballs into the pot. In a bowl, mix the grape jelly, chili sauce, spices and water and then combine.

2. Pour the mixture into the pot and stir. Cover and lock the lid.

3. Set to cook on high pressure for 10 minutes and then quick release pressure once ready.

4. Let the meatballs cool. After that, serve and garnish with green onions.

Nutrition Information:

Calories 330; Fat 16g; protein 7g ; Net carbs 12g; Fiber 1g; Sugar 2g; Sodium 539mg

17. Garlic Bread

(Total Time: 1 hr | Serves 4)

Ingredients

- Egg white – 3 pieces
- Apple cider vinegar – 2 teaspoons
- Sea salt – 1 teaspoon
- Almond flour - 300ml
- Ground psyllium husk powder – 5 tablespoons
- Baking powder - 2 teaspoons
- Boiling water - 300 ml
- Garlic Butter
- Butter - 110g
- Garlic clove - 1pc
- Fresh parsley chopped – 2 teaspoons
- Salt

Instructions

1. Set the oven at 3500F while mixing the dry ingredients in a bowl.
2. Let the water boil. Add vinegar and egg whites to the bowl and then whisk or stir with a manual mixer for 30 seconds, ensuring that you do not over mix.

3. Using your hands, make 10 pieces rolling them into hot dog buns. Create enough space on the baking sheet to enable expansion.
4. Place in the oven on lower rack and leave to bake for 50 minutes.
5. Prepare garlic butter as the bread is baking by mixing all ingredients together and then place in the fridge.
6. Remove the buns from the oven and let them cool. Remove the garlic butter from the fridge and set aside.
7. Slice the buns in halves and spread the garlic butter on each side and then proceed to bake the bread for 10 minutes.

Nutrition Information:

Calories per serving: 53; Carbohydrates: 5g; Protein: 2g; Fat: 4g; Sugar: 0g; Sodium:98mg; Fiber: 0g

18.   Chocolate Biscuits

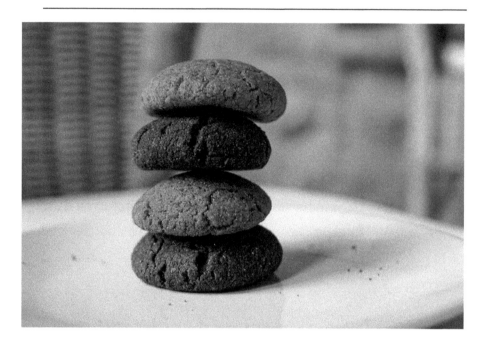

(Total Time: 25 min| Serves 8)

Ingredients

- Whole almonds – 2 cups
- Chia seeds – 2 tablespoons
- Unsweetened shredded coconut – ¼ cup
- Egg – 1
- Coconut oil – 1 cup
- Cacao powder – ¼ cup
- Stevia – 3 tablespoons
- Salt – ¼ teaspoon
- Baking soda – 1 teaspoon

Instructions

1. Get the oven preheated to 3500F.
2. Blend whole almonds and chia seeds into a fairly fine mixture.
3. Have all the ingredients mixed together.
4. Place the mixture on aluminum foil and then refrigerate for about 30 minutes.
5. Cut the dough into thin biscotti shapes and then bake for about 12 minutes.
6. You can enjoy while warm or let it cool and dry further.

Nutrition Information:

Calories 80; Fat 5g; protein 1g; Net carbs 13g; Fiber 0g; Sugar 1g; Sodium 0g

19.   Whipped Coconut Cream with Berries

(Total time – 15 min| Serves 1)

Ingredients

- Unsweetened full fat coconut milk – 1 can
- Berries of choice
- Dark chocolate (Optional)

Instructions

1. Let coconut milk stay in the fridge overnight for about 12 hours.
2. Scoop the thick part and leave water.
3. Whip with a mixer for about 3 minutes.
4. Mix in the berries.
5. Top the cream with chocolate shavings.
6. Serve and enjoy.

Nutrition Information:

Calories 100; Fat 12g; protein 2g; Net carbs 8g; Fiber 0g; Sugar 2g; Sodium 400mg

20.   Sous Vide Egg Bites

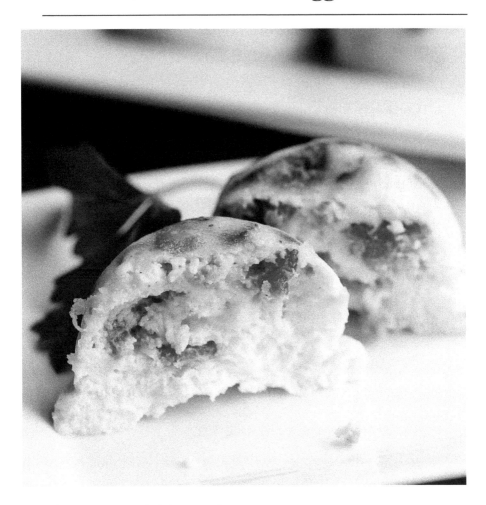

(Total Time: 450 min| Serves 4)

Ingredients

- Large eggs – 4
- Strips of cooked bacon – 4
- Cheddar cheese – ¾ cup

- Heavy cream – ¼ cup
- Cottage cheese – ½ cup

Instructions

1. Set the oven to 3500F.
2. Crack eggs into a blender. Add cottage cheese and a half cup of cheddar cheese. Pulse until well mixed.
3. Spray the glass bowls with cooking spray and then pour ½ cup of the mixture into bowls. Top it up with the remaining shredded cheese and bacon.
4. Place the bowls into a baking dish. Fill the baking dish with water.
5. Bake for 35 minutes or until the mixture becomes solid.

Nutrition Information:

Calories 120; Fat 9g; protein 3g; Net carbs 9g; Fiber 0g; Sugar 2g; Sodium 0mg

21.   Pepperoni Chips

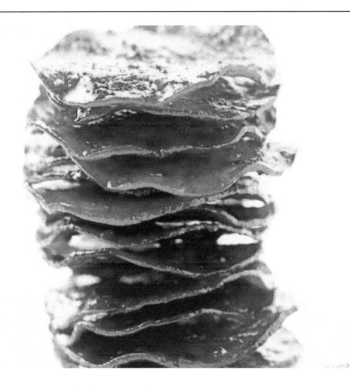

(Total Time: 20 min| Serves 4)

Ingredients

- Pepperoni – 4 oz
- Instructions
- Turn the oven to broil and then line the baking sheet with parchment paper.

Instructions

1. Place pepperoni slices in a single layer. Bake for 2 minutes and watch as they brown in the edges.
2. Remove from the oven. Transfer to a tray and allow to cool for 10 minutes.
3. Serve and enjoy.

Nutrition Information:

Calories per serving: 96; Carbohydrates: 1g; Protein: 6g; Fat: 8g; Sugar: 0g; Sodium:48mg; Fiber: 0g

22. Cheddar Basil Bites

(Total Time 50 min| Serves 24)

Ingredients

- Heavy whipping cream – 2 tablespoons
- Butter – 6 tablespoons
- Shredded cheddar cheese – 1cup
- Coconut flour – ¼ cup
- Grated parmesan cheese – ¼ cup
- Fresh basil – 2 tablespoon

Instructions

1. Get the oven preheated to 3250F and then line two baking sheets with parchment paper.
2. Place butter in a medium bowl. Add heavy cream and combine.
3. Add parmesan cheese, cheddar cheese and coconut flour and then combine using a spatula.
4. Fold in basil and use your hand to incorporate the mixture.
5. Place parchment paper over the counter and then roll the mixture out to about ¼ inch thick. Use a cookie cutter to cut the 24 pieces of crackers. After that, place the crackers on the baking dish.
6. Bake for 15 minutes and check towards the end to ensure you don't overcook them.

Nutrition Information:

Calories per serving: 58; Carbohydrates: 0.5g; Protein: 2g; Fat: 5g; Sugar: 0g; Sodium:78mg; Fiber: 0g

23.   Zucchini Chips

(Total Time: 25min| Serves 4)

Ingredients

- Organic zucchini – 1 pound
- Olive oil – 1/3 cup
- Unrefined sea salt to taste

Instructions

1. Trim the ends of zucchini and then thinly slice them.
2. Oil a microwave safe plate with olive oil and then place zucchini slices. Spray with olive oil and unrefined sea salt to taste.
3. Cook for 10 minutes uncovered. Check the chips. Cook for more minutes until crispy.
4. Allow to cool and then serve with dressings and dips of your choice.

Nutrition Information:

Calories 290; Fat 27g; protein 4g; Net carbs 7g; Fiber 1g; Sugar 1g; Sodium 210mg

24.   Easy Almond Butter Fat Bombs

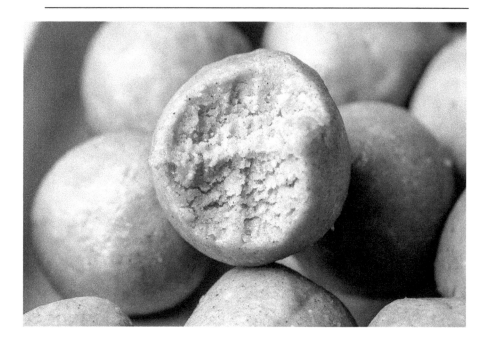

(Total Time: 10 min| Serves 6)

Ingredients

- Almond butter – ¼ cup
- Unrefined coconut oil – ¼ cup
- Cacao powder – 2 tablespoons
- Erythritol – ¼ cup

Instructions

1. Mix almond butter and coconut together in a bowl. Microwave for about 45 minutes and then stir until smooth.
2. Stir in cacao powder and erythritol and then pour into silicone molds.

3. Refrigerate until firm.

Nutrition Information:

Calories per serving: 189; Carbohydrates: 3g; Protein: 3g; Fat: 19g; Sugar: 0g; Sodium:220mg; Fiber: 2g

25. Greek Orange Honey Cake with Pistachios

(Total Time: 30 min| Serves 6)

Ingredients

- Large eggs – 5
- Low fat Greek yoghurt – 1 cup
- Granulated sugar – 2 cups
- Ground almonds – 5 tablespoons
- Zest of lemon – 1
- All-purpose flour – 1 ¼ cup
- Course semolina – 1 cup
- Baking powder – 2 teaspoons
- Virgin olive oil -3/4 cup
- Shaved almonds for topping (optional)
- Honey Pistachio Syrup
- Shelled salted pistachios – 1 ¼ cup
- Honey – 1 ¼ cup
- Orange juice – 2
- Lemon juice – 1

Instructions

1. Get the oven preheated to 3500F. Grease the baking dish with butter and dust with flour and then shake the pan to evenly coat it with flour.

2. Place ingredients for the cake into a mixing bowl and then whisk to combine. Pour butter into the prepared baking pan and then spread the mixture evenly using a spatula.

3. Bake in the oven for 30 minutes or until golden and cooked through. Remove from the oven once ready. Set aside to cool.

4. Once the cake has cooled, prepare the honey syrup by toasting pistachio into a non-stick pan and then place over medium heat.

5. Stir in honey once it begins to smell and then add orange and lemon juice. Bring to a boil for about 2 minutes or until syrupy.

6. Stab some holes into the cake to create holes. Pour honey pistachio syrup over the cake evenly.

7. Sprinkle the shaved almonds as desired.

8. Cut the cake to squares. Serve and enjoy.

Nutrition information:

Calories per serving: 352; Carbohydrates: 58g; Protein: 8g; Fat: 10g; Sugar: 32g; Sodium:30mg; Fiber: 3g

26.   Avocado Chips

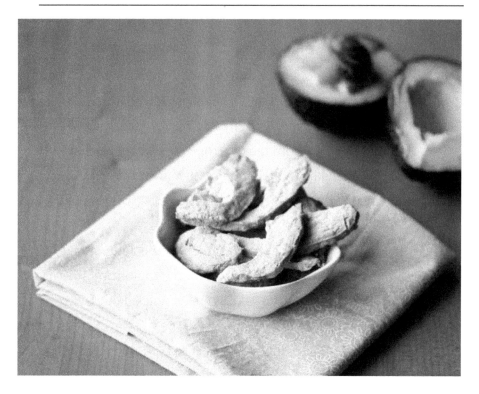

(Total Time: 30 min| Serves 4)

Ingredients

- Large ripe avocado – 1
- Freshly grated parmesan – ¾ cup
- Lemon juice – 1 teaspoon
- Garlic powder – ½ teaspoon
- Kosher salt
- Italian seasoning – ½ teaspoon
- Freshly ground black pepper

Instructions

1. Get the oven preheated to 3250F and then line the baking dish with parchment paper.
2. In a bowl, mash avocado and then stir in parmesan, lemon juice, garlic powder, salt, pepper and Italian seasoning.
3. Place scoops of the mixture on the baking sheet and leave space of 3" apart between each scoop.
4. Place in the oven and bake until crisp and golden or for 15 minutes.
5. Remove from the oven and then allow to cool.
6. Serve while at room temperature.

Nutrition Information:

Calories per serving: 160; Carbohydrates: 17g; Protein: 2g; Fat: 3g; Sugar: 0g; Sodium:

12mg; Fiber: 3g

27. Pepperoni Pizza Mozzarella Crisps

(Total Time: 15 min| Serves 4)

Ingredients

- Shredded mozzarella cheese – ½ cup
- Diced pepperoni
- Garlic powder – 1 teaspoon

Instructions

1. Get the oven preheated to 350oF and then line the cookie sheet in parchment paper.
2. Place mozzarella onto the parchment paper and spread it slightly in a circle.
3. Sprinkle mozzarella with garlic powder and basil and then top with pieces of chopped pepperoni.
4. Place in the oven and allow to bake for 6 minutes or until the edges of the cheese turn golden brown.
5. Remove from the oven. Allow to cool.
6. Enjoy with your preferred dip.

Nutrition information:

Calories per serving: 158; Carbohydrates: 18g; Protein: 20g; Fat: 18g; Sugar: 0g; Sodium:420mg; Fiber: 0g

28. Parmesan Crisps

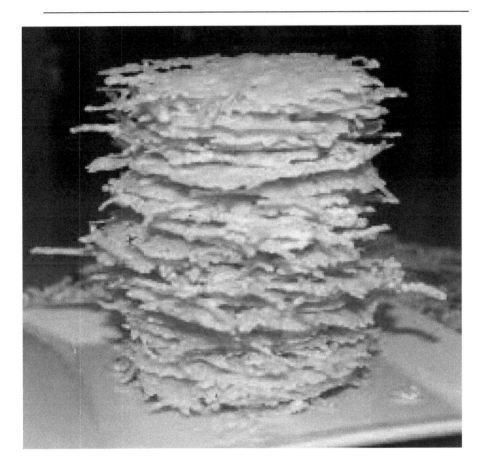

(Total Time: 20 min | Serves 2)

Ingredients

- Grated parmesan cheese – 8 tablespoons
- Provolone cheese – 2 slices
- Medium jalapeno – 1

Instructions

1. On a parchment paper, place eight mounds of parmesan cheese an inch apart from one another.
2. Slice the jalapeno and then lay on the parchment paper. Bake at 4250F for about 5 minutes.
3. Remove from the oven. Allow to cool and then lay each one onto a mound of parmesan as you slightly press it down.
4. Split each of the provolone slice into pieces and then place over jalapeno and parmesan.
5. Let it bake for 5 more minutes. After that, remove and allow to cool.

Nutrition Information:

Calories per serving: 162; Carbohydrates: 1.5g; Protein: 14g; Fat: 10g; Sugar: 1g; Sodium:200mg; Fiber: 0g

29. Toasted Spicy Almonds

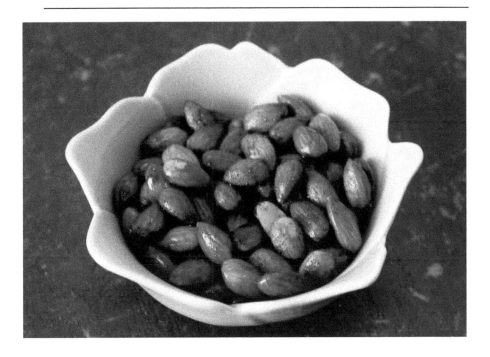

(Total Time: 1 hr 10 min| Serves 6)

- Ingredients
- Almonds – 4 cups
- Butter – 2 tablespoons
- Ground cinnamon – 1 teaspoon
- Vanilla extract – 1 tablespoon
- Egg whites – 2
- Salt - 1 teaspoon

Instructions

1. Get the oven preheated to 4500F.
2. Add all ingredients apart from almonds into a bowl and then stir until well combined.
3. Add almonds to the mixture and then combine until well coated.
4. Transfer the mixture into a baking pan. Allow to bake for about 10 minutes as you stir occasionally.
5. Remove from the oven once ready. Allow to cool before serving.

Nutrition information:

Calories per serving: 350; Carbohydrates: 9g; Protein: 11g; Fat: 7g; Sugar: 0g; Sodium:356mg; Fiber: 5g

30.   Tomato Basil Skewers

(Total Time: 20 min| Serves 4)

Ingredients

- Fresh mozzarella balls – 16
- Fresh basil leaves – 16
- Cherry tomatoes – 16
- Olive oil to drizzle
- Salt and freshly ground pepper

Instructions

Thread mozzarella, tomatoes and basil on a small skewer and then drizzle with oil and sprinkle with salt and pepper.

Nutrition information:

Calories per serving: 46; Carbohydrates: 1g; Protein: 3g; Fat: 3g; Sugar: 0g; Sodium:217mg; Fiber: 1g

31.   Cold Feta Olive Spread

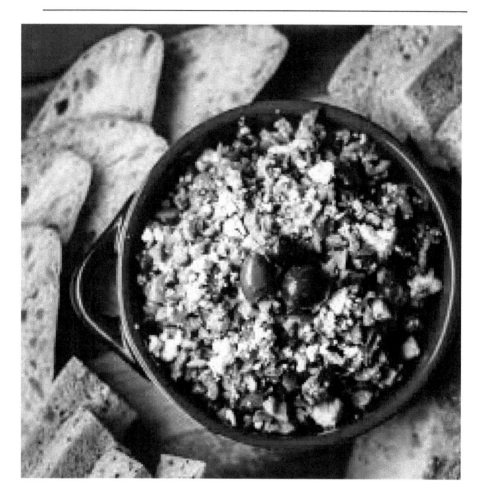

PREPARATION TIME: 24 hours

Ingredients:

- cup olives, pitted, sliced ¼ cup feta, diced
- 1 tbsp extra-virgin olive oil
- 1 clove garlic, crushed
- 1 tsp chopped rosemary

- Juice and zest of half a whole lemon
- Pinch of ground pepper and crushed red pepper

Directions:

1. Combine all ingredients in a bowl with lid. Mix well.
2. Cover and refrigerate for up to 24 hours.
3. Serve as toppings for your choice of crackers or baguette for snacks.

Per 2 tbsp serving: 73 calories, 7g total fat, 2g sat, 4g monosaturated, 6g cholesterol, 263mg sodium, 2g total carbohydrates, 1g dietary fibre, 14mg potassium, 1g protein

32.   Fun Picnic Snack

PREPARATION TIME: 5 minutes

Ingredients:

- slices whole-wheat bread 12 pcs. olives, cured in oil 20 pcs. cherry tomatoes
- ½ cup aged cheese, cubed

Directions:

1. Arrange all ingredients on your favourite platter and serve.

Per serving: 201 calories, 11g total fat, 3.5g sat, 1g monosaturated, 8g cholesterol, 693mg sodium, 23g total carbohydrates, 4g dietary fibre, 474mg potassium, 7g protein

33.   Creamy Blueberry

PREPARATION TIME: 2 hours and 5 minutes

Ingredients:

- cup reduced-fat cream cheese ¼ cup low-fat plain Greek yogurt 1 cup fresh blueberries
- 1 tsp freshly grated lemon zest
- 1 tsp honey

Directions:

1. In a medium bowl, break up cream cheese using a fork. Add yogurt and honey.
2. Using an electric mixer, beat at high speed until mixture is creamy. Stir in lemon zest.
3. Per serving: 156 calories, 7g total fat, 4g sat, 0g monosaturated, 22g cholesterol, 151mg sodium, 19g total carbohydrates, 2g dietary fibre, 189mg potassium, 6g protein

34.   Cherries in Ricotta

PREPARATION TIME: 5 minutes

Ingredients:

- 1 ½ cups cherries, pitted
- ¼ cup part-skim ricotta
- 2 tbsp toasted slivered almonds

Directions:

In a bowl, place cherries and microwave until warm. Top with ricotta and almonds.

Per serving: 133 calories.

35.   Mediterranean Spinach Cakes

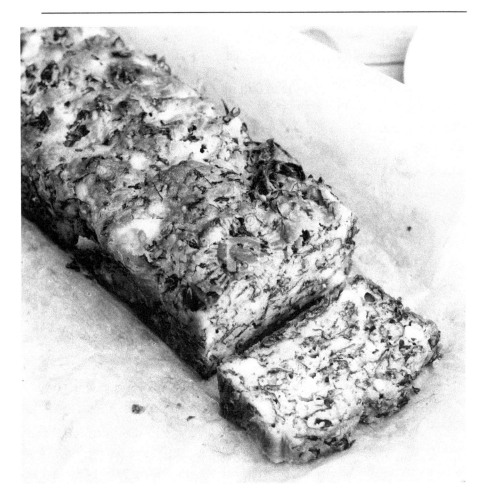

PREPARATION TIME: 10 minutes

COOKING TIME: 20 minutes

Ingredients:

- ¾ cup fresh spinach
- cup finely shredded Parmesan cheese 6 ¼ cup low-fat cottage cheese
- 1 egg, beaten
- ½ a clove garlic, minced Salt and pepper

Directions:

1. Preheat oven to 400 degrees F.
2. In a food processor, pulse spinach until finely chopped then place in a bowl. Add in cottage cheese, Parmesan, garlic, egg, salt and pepper. Mix well.
3. Spray muffin cooking pan with a healthy cooking spray (olive oil is great). Add in spinach mixture.
4. Bake for 20 minutes. Let it stand for 5 minutes. Place muffins in a serving plate. Sprinkle with parmesan if desired.
5. Serve.

Per 2 serving: 141 calories, 8g total fat, 4g sat, 3g monosaturated, 123g cholesterol, 456mg sodium, 6g total carbohydrates, 2g dietary fibre, 560mg potassium, 13g protein

36.　Creamy Lentil Cakes

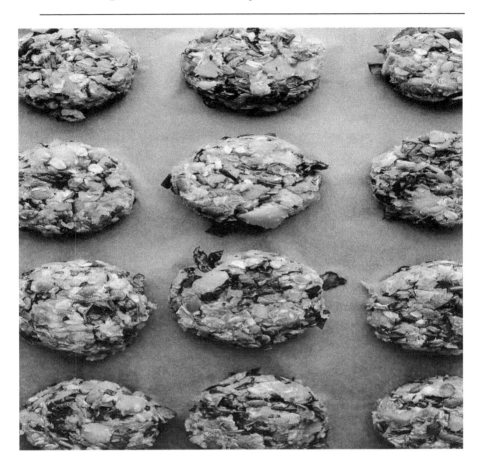

PREPARATION TIME: 10 minutes

COOKING TIME: 10 minutes

Ingredients:

- 1 cup cooked lentils
- 1 whole egg and 1 egg white
- ¼ cup breadcrumbs

- 4 tbsp reduced fat sour cream
- 1 tbsp olive oil
- 1 jalapeno, minced
- 1 clove garlic, minced
- 2 tbsp diced carrot
- 1 tbsp chopped cilantro
- Juice of 1 lime
- 1 tbsp and 1 tsp cumin
- salt

Directions:

1. Heat olive oil in a skillet, sauté onion, jalapeno, garlic and carrots for about 3-4 minutes. Switch off heat.
2. In a bowl, combine cooked lentils and sautéed mixture. Add eggs, breadcrumbs, cumin and chopped cilantro. Combine thoroughly.
3. Form patties from the mixture and fry in the skillet for 2 minutes on each side on medium high heat. Place aside.
4. In a small bowl, combine sour cream, lime juice and 1 tsp cumin.
5. Arrange the lentil cakes on a bed of spinach and top with the sour cream dressing. Serve and enjoy.

37.   Roasted Squash Wrap

PREPARATION TIME: 15 minutes

COOKING TIME: 30 minutes

Ingredients:

- 4 wedges Kabocha squash, about 2cm thick each ½ cup cubed cucumber
- Half a whole avocado, mashed
- 4 leaves Swiss chard
- 1 tbsp olive oil
- Salt and pepper to taste

Directions:

1. Preheat oven to 425 degrees F.
2. Slice squash into wedges and toss with oil and sprinkle with pepper and salt. Place in a baking tray and bake for 15 minutes. Flip each squash and cook for another 15 minutes. Place aside.
3. Lay collard flat, place a squash wedge in the middle and smear an avocado on top of the squash, sprinkle with salt and pepper and top with cucumber slices. Roll and serve.

38.   Olive Feta-honey Cakes

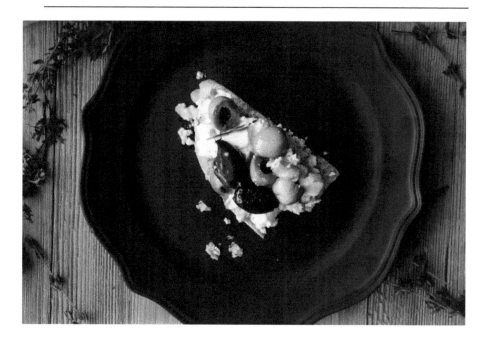

PREPARATION TIME: 5 minutes

COOKING TIME: 25 minutes

Ingredients:

- cup ground almonds
- cup feta cheese
- cup sugar
- 1 tbsp honey
- 3 tbsp extra virgin olive oil
- cup flour
- tsp baking powder ¼ cup olives, halved 2 tbsp brown sugar

Directions:

1. Preheat oven to 347 degrees F.
2. In a mixer, process cheese, honey and sugar until a smooth texture is achieved. Pour in the olive oil.
3. In another bowl, combine flour, baking powder and almonds. Combine with the cheese mixture.
4. Divide batter among greased cake molds and top each with olive oil and brown sugar. Bake for 25 minutes. Serve.

39.   Hazelnut Cookies

PREPARATION TIME: 10 minutes

COOKING TIME: 30 minutes

Ingredients:

- cup and 2 tbsp sugar 2 egg whites
- 1 cup toasted hazelnuts, skinned Pinch of salt
- tsp vanilla extract

Directions:

1. Preheat oven to 325 degrees Fahrenheit with a rack close to the oven's centre. Prepare a parchment paper lined baking sheet.
2. In a food processor, pulse nuts and sugar until finely ground and scrape into a large bowl.
3. Using an electric mixer, beat egg whites and salt in a bowl on high speed until stiff peaks form.
4. Using a rubber spatula, gently fold egg whites into nut mixture. Add vanilla and mix until combined.
5. Pour batter using tablespoon with 2 inches apart on the prepared baking sheets. Bake until golden brown switching the pans back to front and top to bottom halfway for 30 minutes. Let it cool for 5 minutes before serving.

Per cookie serving: 88 calories, 5g total fat, 0g sat, 4g monosaturated, 0g cholesterol, 46mg sodium, 10g total carbohydrates, 1g dietary fibre, 61mg potassium, 2g protein

40.   Feta-Olive Cakes

PREPARATION TIME: 15 minutes

COOKING TIME: 25 minutes

Ingredients:

- 6 tbsp powdered sugar
- 3 tbsp ground almonds
- ½ cup all purpose flour
- cup extra virgin olive oil 2 tbsp crumbled feta cheese 1 tbsp honey
- ½ tsp baking powder
- cup pitted Kalamata olives, halved 1 tbsp sugar

Directions:

1. Preheat oven to 350 degrees Fahrenheit.
2. In a mixer, process cheese, sugar and honey until smooth. Add olive oil.
3. In a bowl, combine flour, ground almonds and baking powder. Combine to the cheese mixture while mixing.
4. Pour batter into greased muffin pans and top with half an olive. Sprinkle top with brown sugar and bake for 25 minutes until lightly brown.

41.   Root Vegetable Pave

Total Time Prep: 40 min. Bake: 1-3/4 hours + standing

Ingredients

- 3 medium russet potatoes, peeled
- 2 large carrots
- 2 medium turnips, peeled
- 1 large onion, halved
- 1 medium fennel bulb, fronds reserved
- 1/2 cup all-purpose flour
- 1 cup heavy whipping cream
- 1 tablespoon minced fresh thyme, plus more for topping
- 1 tablespoon minced fresh rosemary
- 1/2 teaspoon salt
- 1/2 teaspoon pepper, plus more for topping
- 1 cup shredded Asiago cheese, divided

HOW TO MAKE IT

1. Preheat oven to 350°. With a mandoline or vegetable peeler, cut the first 5 ingredients into very thin slices. Transfer to a large bowl; toss with flour. Stir in the cream, thyme, 1 tablespoon rosemary, salt and pepper.

2. Place half of the vegetable mixture into a greased 9-in. springform pan. Sprinkle with 1/2 cup cheese. Top with remaining vegetable mixture. Place pan on a baking sheet and cover with a double thickness of foil.

3. Bake until vegetables are tender and easily pierced with a knife, 1-3/4 to 2 hours.

4. Remove from oven and top foil with large canned goods as weights. Let stand 1 hour. Remove cans, foil and rim from pan before cutting. Top with remaining cheese.

5. Add reserved fennel fronds and, as desired, additional fresh thyme and pepper. Refrigerate leftovers.

Nutritional Information

1 slice: 248 calories, 15g fat (9g saturated fat), 46mg cholesterol, 216mg sodium, 23g carbohydrate (4g sugars, 2g fiber), 7g protein.

42. Spinach And Artichoke Pizza

Total Time Prep: 25 min. Bake: 20 min.

Ingredients

- 1-1/2 to 1-3/4 cups white whole wheat flour
- 1-1/2 teaspoons baking powder
- 1/4 teaspoon salt
- 1/4 teaspoon each dried basil, oregano and parsley flakes
- 3/4 cup beer or nonalcoholic beer

TOPPINGS:

- 1-1/2 teaspoons olive oil
- 1 garlic clove, minced
- 2 cups shredded Italian cheese blend
- 2 cups fresh baby spinach
- 1 can (14 ounces) water-packed quartered artichoke hearts, drained and coarsely chopped
- 2 medium tomatoes, seeded and coarsely chopped
- 2 tablespoons thinly sliced fresh basil

HOW TO MAKE IT

1. Preheat oven to 425°. In a large bowl, whisk 1-1/2 cups flour, baking powder, salt and dried herbs until blended. Add beer, stirring just until moistened.

2. Turn dough onto a well-floured surface; knead gently 6-8 times, adding more flour if needed. Press dough to fit a greased 12-in. pizza pan.
3. Pinch edge to form a rim. Bake until edge is lightly browned, about 8 minutes.
4. Mix oil and garlic; spread over crust. Sprinkle with 1/2 cup cheese; layer with spinach, artichoke hearts and tomatoes.
5. Sprinkle with remaining cheese.
6. Bake until crust is golden and cheese is melted, 8-10 minutes. Sprinkle with fresh basil.

NUTRITIONAL INFORMATION

1 slice: 290 calories, 10g fat (6g saturated fat), 27mg cholesterol, 654mg sodium, 32g carbohydrate (1g sugars, 5g fiber), 14g protein. Diabetic Exchanges: 2 starch, 1 medium-fat meat, 1 vegetable.

43.   Breadstick Pizza

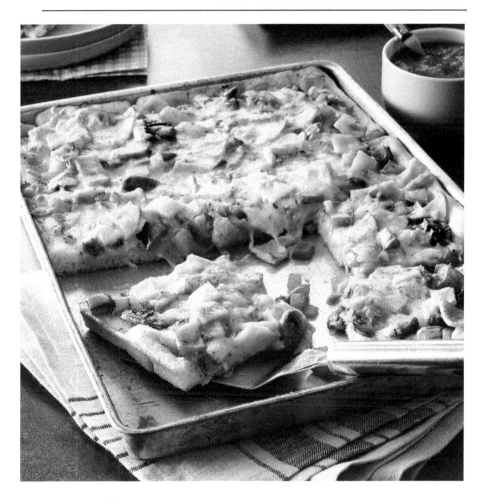

Prep: 25 min. Bake: 20 min.

INGREDIENTS

- 2 tubes (11 ounces each) refrigerated breadsticks
- 1/2 pound sliced fresh mushrooms
- 2 medium green peppers, chopped

- 1 medium onion, chopped
- 1-1/2 teaspoons Italian seasoning, divided
- 4 teaspoons olive oil, divided
- 1-1/2 cups shredded cheddar cheese, divided
- 5 ounces Canadian bacon, chopped
- 1-1/2 cups shredded part-skim mozzarella cheese
- Marinara sauce

HOW TO MAKE IT

1. Unroll breadsticks into a greased 15x10x1-in. baking pan. Press onto the bottom and up the sides of pan; pinch seams to seal. Bake at 350° until set, 6-8 minutes.

2. Meanwhile, in a large skillet, saute the mushrooms, peppers, onion and 1 teaspoon Italian seasoning in 2 teaspoons oil until crisp-tender; drain.

3. Brush crust with remaining oil. Sprinkle with 3/4 cup cheddar cheese; top with vegetable mixture and Canadian bacon. Combine mozzarella cheese and remaining cheddar cheese; sprinkle over top. Sprinkle with remaining Italian seasoning.

4. Bake until cheese is melted and crust is golden brown, 20-25 minutes. Serve with marinara sauce.

5. Freeze option: Bake crust as directed, add toppings and cool. Securely wrap and freeze unbaked pizza. To use, unwrap pizza; bake as directed, increasing time as necessary.

NUTRITIONAL INFORMATION

1 piece (calculated without marinara sauce): 267 calories, 11g fat (6g saturated fat), 27mg cholesterol, 638mg sodium, 29g carbohydrate (5g sugars, 2g fiber), 13g protein.

44.   **Summer Dessert Pizza**

Total Time

Prep: 35 min. + chilling Bake: 15 min. + cooling

INGREDIENTS

- 1/4 cup butter, softened
- 1/2 cup sugar
- 1 large egg
- 1/4 teaspoon vanilla extract
- 1/4 teaspoon lemon extract
- 1-1/4 cups all-purpose flour
- 1/4 teaspoon baking powder
- 1/4 teaspoon baking soda
- 1/4 teaspoon salt

GLAZE:

- 1/4 cup sugar
- 2 teaspoons cornstarch
- 1/4 cup water
- 1/4 cup orange juice
- TOPPING:
- 4 ounces cream cheese, softened
- 1/4 cup confectioners' sugar
- 1 cup whipped topping
- 1 firm banana, sliced

- 1 cup sliced fresh strawberries
- 1 can (8 ounces) mandarin oranges, drained
- 2 kiwifruit, peeled and thinly sliced
- 1/3 cup fresh blueberries

HOW TO MAKE IT

1. In a small bowl, cream butter and sugar until light and fluffy. Beat in egg and extracts. Combine flour, baking powder, baking soda and salt; add to creamed mixture and beat well. Cover and refrigerate for 30 minutes.
2. Press dough into a greased 12- to 14-in. pizza pan. Bake at 350° for 12-14 minutes or until light golden brown. Cool completely on a wire rack.
3. For glaze, combine sugar and cornstarch in a small saucepan. Stir in the water and orange juice until smooth. Bring to a boil; cook and stir for 1-2 minutes or until thickened. Cool to room temperature, about 30 minutes.
4. For topping, in a small bowl, beat cream cheese and confectioners' sugar until smooth. Add whipped topping; mix well. Spread over crust. Arrange fruit on top. Brush glaze over fruit. Store in the refrigerator.
5. Test Kitchen Tips
6. Use premade sugar cookie dough to save a bit of time.
7. If you're in a pinch, orange marmalade works in place of the glaze.

NUTRITIONAL INFORMATION

1 piece: 176 calories, 7g fat (4g saturated fat), 29mg cholesterol, 118mg sodium, 27g carbohydrate (17g sugars, 1g fiber), 2g protein.

45.   Patriotic Taco Salad

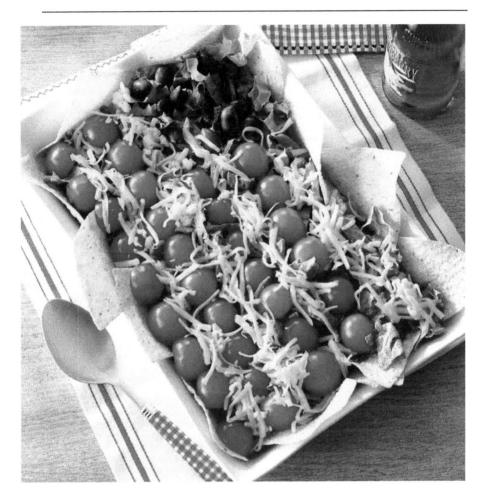

Total Time Prep: 10 min. Cook: 20 min.

INGREDIENTS

- 1 pound ground beef
- 1 medium onion, chopped
- 1-1/2 cups water

- 1 can (6 ounces) tomato paste
- 1 envelope taco seasoning
- 6 cups tortilla or corn chips
- 4 to 5 cups shredded lettuce
- 9 to 10 pitted large olives, sliced lengthwise
- 2 cups Kerrygold shredded cheddar cheese
- 2 cups cherry tomatoes, halved

HOW TO MAKE IT

1. In a large skillet, cook beef and onion over medium heat until meat is no longer pink; drain. Stir in the water, tomato paste and taco seasoning. Bring to a boil. Reduce heat; simmer, uncovered, for 20 minutes.
2. Place chips in an ungreased 13x9-in. dish. Spread beef mixture evenly over the top. Cover with lettuce. For each star, arrange five olive slices together in the upper left corner. To form stripes, add cheese and tomatoes in alternating rows. Serve immediately.
3. Editor's Note: If you wish to prepare this salad in advance, omit the layer of chips and serve them with the salad.

NUTRITIONAL INFORMATION

1 cup: 357 calories, 20g fat (9g saturated fat), 63mg cholesterol, 747mg sodium, 24g carbohydrate (4g sugars, 2g fiber), 20g protein.

46. KALE BRUSCHETTA

Ready In: 25 minutes

INGREDIENTS

- 1 bunch kale
- 1 loaf fresh 100% whole-grain bread, sliced
- ½ cup Cannellini Bean Sauce
- 1 cup grape tomatoes, halved
- balsamic glaze

HOW TO MAKE IT

1. Place the kale leaves in a large pot of boiling water. Cover and cook until tender, about 5 minutes. Drain in a colander, then squeeze out any extra liquid with your hands (you don't want soggy bread).

2. Toast 8 pieces of bread, and place them on a handsome serving platter.

3. Spread a tablespoon of the Cannellini Bean Sauce on the toasted bread, then cover with a layer of kale and top with a scattering of grape tomatoes. Drizzle generously with the balsamic glaze, and grab one for yourself before they all disappear.

47. Caramelized Onion & Pepper Vegan Quesadillas

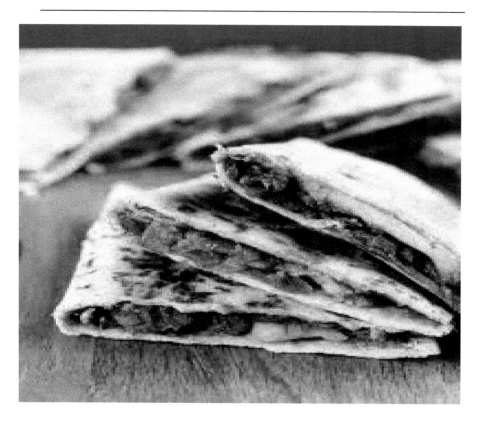

Prep-time: 2 hours 15 minutes / Cook Time: 15 minutes

INGREDIENTS

- ¾ cup raw cashews, soaked for 2 hours
- ½ cup nutritional yeast flakes
- 1 lime, juiced
- ½ tablespoon stoneground mustard, no-salt added
- ½ cup water

- 1 yellow onion, sliced thin
- 1 red bell pepper, sliced thin
- 1 yellow bell pepper, sliced thin
- 1½ tablespoons ground cumin
- 1½ teaspoon chili powder
- 8 100% corn tortillas, no salt or oil added
- 2 cups fresh spinach, loosely packed

HOW TO MAKE IT

1. Make the cheese sauce: Add the cashews, nutritional yeast, lime, stoneground mustard and water to a blender. Blend until it the sauce is creamy. Set it aside.

2. Make the onion-pepper filling: Place a sauté pan over medium heat. Add the sliced onion and bell pepper. Stir in the cumin and chili powder. Cover and cook for 5 minutes, stirring occasionally so the veggies don't stick to the bottom of the pan. Then stir in a tablespoon of water and continue cooking uncovered. When the water evaporates stir in another tablespoon of water, continuing to sauté until the onions are caramelized.

3. Turn the heat to low. Pour the cheese sauce into the onion and peppers. Stir well and then cover with a lid so the mixture doesn't dry out.

4. Make the first quesadilla: Place a non-stick pan over medium heat. Let it heat for 5 minutes. Then place one of the tortillas into the pan. Set a timer, letting the first side toast for 2 minutes and then flip. Set the timer for another 2 minutes. As

you wait, carefully scoop about ¼ of the filling onto the tortilla and spread it evenly, forming a single layer of peppers and onions. Layer ½ cup of spinach across the onions and peppers. Place the second tortilla on top of the spinach.

5. Once the timer goes off or the bottom side is toasted, use a large spatula to carefully flip the entire quesadilla. Toast the second tortilla for 2-3 minutes.

6. When the quesadilla is done transfer it to a plate. Repeat this process with the remaining filling to make a total of 4 quesadillas. Note that subsequent quesadillas may require less cooking time because the pan will be hotter. You may want to turn the heat down slightly after the first couple. Slice the quesadillas into triangular pieces and serve.

7. Chef's Note: Soaking the cashews softens them so they become creamy when blended. If you're using a high-powered blender such as a vitamix, the nuts do not need to be soaked.

48.   Waffled Falafel

Prep Time: 20 minutes

Ingredients:

- 2 Large Egg Whites
- 2 cans of Garbanzo Beans
- 1 1/2 tablespoons of All Purpose Flour
- 1/4 cup of Chopped Fresh Parsley

- 1 Chopped Medium Onion
- 1/4 cup of Chopped Fresh Cilantro
- 3 Cloves of Roasted Garlic
- 1/4 teaspoon of Cayenne Pepper
- 2 teaspoons of Ground Cumin
- 1 teaspoon of Ground Coriander
- 1/4 teaspoon of Ground Black Pepper
- 1 3/4 teaspoons of Salt
- Pinch of Ground Cardamom
- Cooking Spray

Directions:

1. Preheat your waffle iron. Spray inside of your iron with your cooking spray.

2. Process your garbanzo beans in your food processor until they are coarsely

chopped.

3. Add in your egg whites, cilantro, onion, parsley, cumin, flour, coriander, garlic,

salt, black pepper, cayenne pepper, and ground cardamom to your garbanzo beans.

4. Pulse in your food processor until your batter resembles a coarse meal. Scrap

down the sides while pulsing.

5. Pour your batter into your bowl and stir it with your fork.

6. Spoon 1/4 cup of batter onto each section of your waffle iron. Cook until they are

evenly browned. Should take approximately 5 minutes. Repeat the process with

your batter until it has all been used.

7. Serve!

49.　Artichokes Alla Romana (Serves 8)

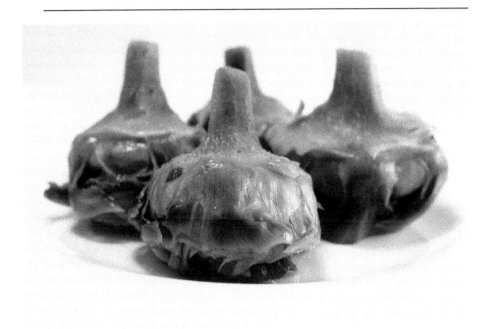

Prep Time: 40 minutes

Ingredients:

- 4 Large Artichokes
- 1/3 cup of Grated Parmesan Cheese
- 2 cups of Fresh Whole-Wheat Breadcrumbs
- 2 tablespoons of Finely Chopped Flat-Leaf Parsley
- 1 cup + 3 tablespoons of Vegetable Stock
- 1 tablespoon of Olive Oil
- 2 Halved Lemons
- 1 tablespoon of Grated Lemon Zest

- 3 cloves of Finely Chopped Garlic
- 1 teaspoon of Chopped Fresh Oregano
- 1 cup of Dry White Wine
- 1 tablespoon of Minced Shallot
- 1/4 teaspoon of Ground Black Pepper

Directions:

1. Preheat your oven to 400 degrees.

2. In your bowl, combine your olive oil and breadcrumbs. Toss well to coat. Spread

your crumbs in your shallow baking pan and put in your oven, stirring once halfway

through, until your crumbs are lightly golden. Should take approximately 10 min-

utes. Set to the side to cool.

3. Working with 1 artichoke at a time, snap off any of their tough outer leaves and

trim their stem flush with their base. Cut off the top 1/3 of the leaves using a ser-

rated knife, and trim off any of the remaining thorns with your scissors. Rub the cut

edges with your lemon half to prevent discoloration. Separate the inner leaves and pull out any small leaves from the center. Using your melon baller or spoon, scoop

out the fuzzy choke, then squeeze some of your lemon juice into the cavity. Trim all

your remaining artichokes in the same exact manner.

3. In your large-sized bowl, toss your breadcrumbs with your Parmesan, garlic, pep-

per, lemon zest, and parsley. Add your 3 tablespoons of vegetable stock, 1 table-

spoon at a time, using just enough for your stuffing to begin sticking together in

smaller clumps.

4. Using 2/3 of your stuffing, mound it slightly in the center of your artichokes.

Then, starting at the bottom, spread the leaves open and spoon a rounded teaspoon

of your stuffing near the base of each leaf. (The artichokes can be prepared to this

point hours ahead and kept refrigerated.)

5. In your Dutch oven with a tight fit lid, combine your 1 cup of vegetable stock,

shallot, oregano, and wine. Bring to a boil, then reduce your heat to low. Arrange

your artichokes, stem end down, in the liquid in a single layer. Cover and simmer

until all your outer leaves are tender. Should take approximately 45 minutes (add

more water if necessary).

6. Transfer your artichokes to your rack and allow it to cool slightly. Cut each of

your artichokes into quarters.

50.   Mediterranean Wrap

Ingredients

- Ingredient Checklist
- 1 red onion, sliced
- 1 zucchini, sliced
- 1 eggplant, sliced
- ¼ pound fresh mushrooms, sliced
- 1 red bell pepper, sliced
- 1 tablespoon olive oil
- salt and ground black pepper to taste
- 4 whole grain tortillas
- ¼ cup goat cheese
- ¼ cup basil pesto
- 1 large avocado, sliced

Directions

1. Place the onion, zucchini, eggplant, mushrooms, and bell pepper into a large container with a tight fitting lid. Drizzle the olive oil over the vegetables and season with salt and pepper. Close the lid and shake to coat.

2. Heat a grill pan or skillet over medium heat. Place the seasoned vegetables on the preheated pan, stir and cook until tender, about 10 minutes.

3. Spread each tortilla with 1 tablespoon goat cheese and 1 tablespoon pesto. Divide the sliced avocado among the tortillas

and top with the mixed veggies. Fold in the bottom of each tortilla and roll each up into a snug wrap.

Nutrition Facts

Per Serving: 436 calories; protein 14.6g; carbohydrates 48.4g; fat 26.3g; cholesterol 16.2mg; sodium 433.3mg

51.   Snack Crackers

Prep Time: 65 minutes

Ingredients:

- 1 (1 ounce) package ranch dressing mix
- 1 teaspoon garlic powder
- ½ teaspoon dried dill weed
- ½ cup vegetable oil
- 1 (12 ounce) package oyster crackers

Directions

Mix together ranch dressing mix, garlic powder, dill and vegetable oil. Add crackers and mix gently until the crackers are coated with the mixture. Stir every 10 minutes for 1 hour. Store in an airtight jar.

Nutrition Facts

Per Serving: 217 calories; protein 2.3g; carbohydrates 19.6g; fat 14.2g; sodium 699.1mg. Full Nutrition

52. Furikake Snack Mix

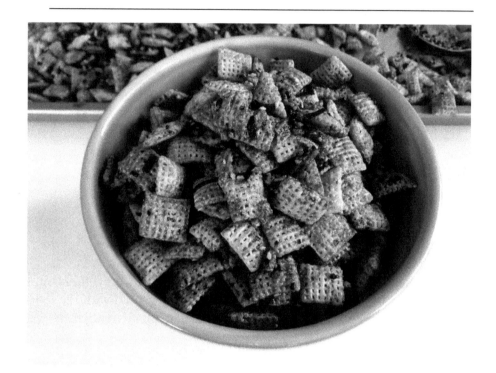

Prep Time: 65 minutes

Ingredients

- Decrease Serving
- 20
- Increase Serving
- Adjust
- Original recipe yields 20 servings
- Ingredient Checklist
- ½ cup butter
- ½ cup white sugar
- ½ cup corn oil

- ½ cup light corn syrup (such as Karo®)
- 2 (12 ounce) packages crispy corn and rice cereal (such as Crispix®)
- 1 (1.9 ounce) container aji nori furikake (seasoned seaweed and sesame rice topping)

Directions

1. Preheat oven to 225 degrees F (110 degrees C).
2. Melt the butter and sugar together in a small sauce pan over low heat. Remove from heat, then stir in the corn oil and corn syrup. Place the cereal on a large baking sheet. Pour the butter mixture over the cereal, then sprinkle the furikake while tossing the cereal to coat.
3. Bake in the preheated oven until the cereal is dry, stirring every 15 minutes to keep cereal from browning too quickly. Allow to cool, then store in an airtight container.

Nutrition Facts

Per Serving: 274 calories; protein 2.5g; carbohydrates 43g; fat 10.7g; cholesterol 12.2mg; sodium 393mg. Full Nutrition

53.   Apple Cheesecake Snack Bars

Time Prep: 30 minutes

Ingredients

- 1 teaspoon butter, or as needed
- Crust:
- 1 ½ cups graham cracker crumbs, or more as needed
- ⅓ cup butter, melted
- Filling:
- 2 (8 ounce) packages cream cheese, at room temperature
- ½ cup white sugar
- 2 large eggs
- 1 teaspoon vanilla extract
- 3 Granny Smith apples - peeled, cored, and diced
- 2 tablespoons white sugar
- ½ teaspoon ground cinnamon
- ¼ teaspoon ground nutmeg
- ¼ teaspoon ground allspice

Streusel:

- ½ cup brown sugar
- ½ cup all-purpose flour
- 1 tablespoon finely chopped walnuts, or to taste (Optional)
- ¼ teaspoon ground cinnamon
- ¼ cup butter, cut into small pieces

Directions:

1. Preheat the oven to 350 degrees F (175 degrees C). Lightly butter a 9x13-inch baking pan.
2. Mix graham cracker crumbs and melted butter together in a bowl until crumbly, adding more crumbs if mixture is too wet. Press crust into the prepared baking pan.
3. Bake in the preheated oven until golden and set, 7 to 8 minutes. Remove from the oven and set aside.
4. Beat cream cheese and 1/2 cup sugar using an electric mixer in a large bowl until smooth. Add eggs, one at a time, beating after each addition. Beat in vanilla extract on low speed until mixture is blended. Pour filling over warm crust.
5. Stir apples, 2 tablespoons sugar, cinnamon, nutmeg, and allspice together in a separate bowl; spoon evenly over filling.
6. Mix brown sugar, flour, walnuts, and cinnamon for streusel together in a bowl. Mix or cut butter into walnut mixture using your fingers or a knife until crumbly. Sprinkle over apple layer.
7. Bake in the preheated oven until cheese filling is set, 30 to 35 minutes.
8. Remove from the oven and let cool completely, about 30 minutes. Cut into small squares and refrigerate until ready to serve

Nutrition Facts

Per Serving: 192 calories; protein 2.7g; carbohydrates 18.6g; fat 12.3g; cholesterol 48.3mg; sodium 127.4mg

Lightning Source UK Ltd.
Milton Keynes UK
UKHW020750030621
384855UK00001B/46